It's Not About the Food

*A Revolutionary Approach To Ending Your
Battle With Food And Finding Freedom From
Overeating*

Alexandra Amor

Copyedit by Jennifer McIntyre
Cover design by Alexandra Amor

Fat Head Publishing
PO Box 916, Ucluelet, BC V0R 3A0
AlexandraAmor.com

Published in Canada with international distribution

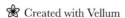 Created with Vellum

Contents

It's Not About the Food

If you, dear reader, are suffering about food,

this book is my gift to you.

Prologue

Every story is a love story.

— Andrew Stanton

I t's 1992. Maybe '93. Davie Street, Vancouver, British Columbia. The basement of a Sheraton hotel. The Pacific Ocean in the form of English Bay is half a block away, glinting like a black mirror, lights from the city reflecting on its onyx surface.

I walk down a flight of wide, carpeted stairs and at the bottom I turn to my right, following the signs. The double doors to a meeting room are propped open, and a woman is sitting behind a table outside the doors in the wide hallway, smiling and registering those who are ahead of me. I wait until it's my turn and then I give my name and contact information. Forms filled out, the woman hands me a packet of information and directs me inside to my first Weight Watchers meeting.

I am 25 years old. And I probably weigh 130 pounds. Max.

In the ensuing years between then and now, there have been countless days when I would have gladly walked across a field of broken glass on my lips if it meant I could weigh 130 pounds again. But on this day in the early '90s I was despondent about that number. It was more than I'd ever weighed. And, in hindsight, the depth of my concern was likely due to the fact that I knew instinctively that number was only going to increase.

Because I felt it constantly: The drive to overeat. It haunted me, following me wherever I went and whatever I did. Shadowing me like I was a princess and it was my personal protection officer. Relentless. Insatiable. And, most frustrating of all, impervious to logic.

I didn't want it. I wanted to be free of the obsessive, needy thoughts I had about food all the time. Why am I like this? I thought to myself, over and over again. Why am I so broken in this way?

Over the ensuing 30 years I tried everything I could think of to fix myself. Talk therapy, what I considered to be healthy diets like Weight Watchers, meditation, self-compassion, emotional freedom technique, hypnosis, and cognitive behavioral therapy. I followed and absorbed everything I could from teachers and leaders in the weight loss field. I went through phases of very restricted eating. And then others that were very permissive. I counted points and calories. Name a self-help book about food and I've probably not only read it but done all the exercises and applied all the external strategies to my life.

None of it worked.

My weight continued to climb, and the drive to overeat dogged me as much as it ever had.

By the time I reached my very late 40s, I had essentially given up on trying to find a solution. I had concluded that I must be broken and unfixable, because, given the amount of effort, energy, and money that I had put into trying to fix myself, and given that the results had thus far been negligible, I'd decided that this was a problem that couldn't be solved. For nearly 30 years I had thrown myself into trying to change, only to discover that change seemed out of my reach.

What I didn't know then, and what I know now, was that the drive I felt to overeat wasn't pointing toward something broken inside me. It wasn't in need of being fixed, and neither was I. It wasn't trying to torture me relentlessly, simply for sport. It was trying to get my attention.

Thankfully, in 2017, I would begin to learn about a new psychological paradigm—the one I'm going to share in this book—and finally, *finally* the drive to overeat would go away.

Once I saw the drive for what it really was, it no longer needed to exist.

I know that likely sounds absurd from where you're sitting, but that, in fact, is one of the core premises of the understanding I'm going to share in this book.

So let's get started.

The Drive to Overeat and Us

If the only thing people learned was not to be afraid of their experience, that alone would change the world.

— Sydney Banks

Welcome.

I'm *so* glad you're here. I feel like we are kindred spirits already. If you've taken the time to read this far, you're likely struggling with an overeating habit, what I sometimes call 'the drive to overeat,' just like I did. And you've probably tried over and over to fix or change that drive.

Me too.

My intention with this book is to open your eyes to a new way of looking at your overeating habit, one that takes a very different approach than the outside-in, willpower-and-deprivation model we're all so used to. I'll explain more about how that works in the next chapter, but for now I wanted to simply say hello.

I know you've been suffering, likely wondering what's wrong with you that you can't put your fork down when you're full or stop going to the cupboard or fridge when you're not even hungry. So I just wanted to say, right up front, that there's nothing wrong with you. There never has been. And throughout this book I'm going to point out why knowing this matters so much to ending your drive to overeat.

You've probably noticed by now that I'm using the phrase 'the drive to overeat' rather than 'food addiction.' For me, the word 'addiction' has a lot of baggage attached to it, so I try to avoid it. I like the way the phrase 'drive to overeat' describes the feeling I experienced. Granted, it's synonymous with the word 'addiction,' but it seems more compassionate and less judgy.

For me, the phrase 'drive to overeat' points to the tension I felt when I wanted to eat in a healthier way and lose weight but experienced a feeling pushing me toward behaviors that I didn't want to participate in like putting more food on my plate than I needed or eating foods that weren't healthy.

But really, 'drive to overeat' and 'addiction' are just words, pointing toward something. Feel free to substitute whatever word or phrase works for you.

Briefly, I'll let you know a little something about me. I'm a writer (obviously) and a coach. Until I wrote this book, I was mostly focused on writing mystery novels, although my first book is an award-winning, Amazon-bestselling memoir about ten years I spent in a cult in the 1990s. (Yes, really.) I'm Canadian and I live on an island off the west coast of British Columbia. I love to read and walk in nature. I'm a quiet person who enjoys a quiet life. The little fishing village I live in is perfectly suited to me this way. At night, with my bedroom window open, the only thing I can hear is the sea lions calling to one another in the inlet near my home.

I struggled with the drive to overeat for my entire adult life, until recently. Despite being a self-help junkie, the understanding I'm going to share here with you is the only thing that's ever made any impact on my struggle to reduce and eliminate the drive I felt to overeat. And as soon as it did, I knew I had to share what I'd seen with others like you.

Housekeeping

Before we dive into the meat of the ideas I'm going to share in this book, I want to address a few things up front.

First, the understanding that I'm going to talk about, commonly called the 3 Principles, or the Inside-Out Understanding, is descriptive, not prescriptive. So reading this book will likely feel very different to any other diet or habit-breaking book you've read.

The prescriptive way of teaching and learning is the one we're likely most familiar with. We encountered it daily in school growing up. We're told what to do, and in what order, which is a fantastic way to learn how to do long division, skateboard, or perform open heart surgery. However, when it comes to living our individual lives as the unique and brilliant humans we each are, it turns out that following someone else's prescription for how to do that can get in our way—for example, when we're trying to understand the drive to overeat.

So, rather than give you a prescriptive list of dos and don'ts or foods to eat and ones to avoid, or techniques for increasing your willpower, I'm going to do a lot of description: describing what's true about you, about your essential nature, and about how all humans work. This might seem counterintuitive to you at first, and possibly even frustrating. But please bear with me.

I remember when a friend turned me on to this understanding back in 2017. I started by reading Michael Neill's book, *The Inside-Out Revolution*. A week or so later my friend asked me how I was getting on with the book, and I said, "It's great. I am enjoying reading it. It's just that…" I paused, thinking about what I felt was missing, "…he hasn't told me what to DO yet." My friend chuckled and said, "That's exactly right. And he's not going to."

Culturally, and especially when it comes to diet and exercise, we're used to being told what to do. We're familiar with being prescribed instructions for how and what and when to eat and exercise. There's an entire industry worth billions of dollars built around this kind of instruction. However, if that approach worked, don't you think it would have, well, *worked* by now? No doubt you've applied nearly endless prescriptions to solving your overeating habit. I know I had before I found this understanding. Did all those lists and rules and instructions work? Not for me. And, in fact, they primarily succeeded in making me feel like a loser and a failure because I couldn't get other people's rules to work for me. What was so broken about me that I couldn't follow a simple food points program?

Nothing, it turns out. Nothing was broken about me, and nothing is broken about you. It's just that applying prescriptive rules to an overeating habit is like trying to change the course of a river by learning to juggle. Your overeating habit doesn't need rules; it needs understanding. So that's what I'm going to offer in this book. I'm going to describe what's really going on, and once you see that, the river will change course on its own.

That might sound like a load of frothy, new-age BS, but I promise you I wouldn't be sharing any of this if I hadn't directly felt and experienced the impact of this understanding myself.

The second bit of housekeeping I want to share is that this book has nothing to do with fat shaming or a lack of body positivity. I firmly believe that all body types are beautiful and that the idealized version of the human body that we're sold (i.e., skinny to the point of emaciation) is unrealistic and, frankly, dangerous. I honestly don't care what you look like or how much you weigh. What really matters to me is how you feel on the inside.

In other words, this book isn't about dieting for dieting's sake. It's actually much deeper than that. We're going to be looking underneath the drive to overeat because that's where the magic lies.

Ask yourself this: Are you at peace? *That's* what I care about. I have not been at peace about food and eating until very recently, until I found and began to explore this understanding. What I recently began to see, and what I want to share with you, is that the peace we seek is inherent to who we are. We *are* peace. And, ironically, that's what the drive to overeat is trying to tell us.

Much of what I'm going to share is based on the awakening experience of a man named Sydney Banks, a Scottish welder and spiritual seeker who lived on an island off the coast of British Columbia (a different island than that one I live on). I never met Syd, but, thankfully, what he shared lives on in the inside-out understanding, and I have learned from many of the people who learned from him.

As you read this book, keep in mind that I'm a person, just like you, muddling through life to the best of my ability. I'm not a doctor of psychology (though I was a psychology major at university). I haven't had an enlightenment experience. What I want to share with you is my very real experience with this understanding, from having been down in the trenches, where you are.

It's sometimes easy to put those who teach, who write books, who have degrees and certificates, on pedestals and assume, perhaps even unconsciously, that they have access to information and awareness that we ourselves don't have. So I want to invite you to not do that with me or with this book. I'm simply sharing what I see about this understanding and how it has positively impacted my life. After trying and failing for 30+ years at so much of the rules-based, outside-in advice that only served to make me more anxious about food, I finally stumbled across this understanding that has made me less anxious about food and eating and weight. Enlightenment and higher learning aren't necessary in order to experience the life-changing effects of this understanding. What I'm going to point toward is innate within you.

Just as Glinda says to Dorothy in the Wizard of Oz, "You've always had the power, my dear."

Now it's time to learn it for yourself.

And finally, learning about this understanding is (possibly) not an overnight solution. In our culture we are so used to instant gratification and immediate results that, it seems to me, we often lose sight of the value of diving deeply into a pursuit or an exploration that isn't necessarily going to offer rewards within half a day of starting.

If you wanted to learn to play an instrument you've never played before, you wouldn't expect to be able to do that in two or three days. You would understand that it would take some time, and that initially it might be frustrating and perhaps also confusing. There would be a new 'language' involved, terms used in the playing of that musical instrument that you've never heard before. Additionally, there would likely be a history and background to that instrument that you don't know but could slowly learn.

Learning about this inside-out understanding is more like learning to play that instrument than it is about instant results; it's not a quick-start diet that promises you'll lose ten pounds in the first week.

When I started following those teachers who talk about this understanding, I was expecting immediate results. I didn't realize that what I was really doing was learning a whole new paradigm about how being human works. It was like learning to play a 12-string guitar without ever having seen one before. I wish I could reach back to the person I was then and say, "Look, this is going to take some time. But the changes you experience will affect your whole life, not just your eating habits. And, when your cascading series of insights tips the balance so that your version of the drive to overeat dissolves, you won't go back to old habits and old fears about food."

This kind of deep and lasting change is worth investing some time in.

You are worth investing time in.

Part One

Your Innate Well-being

Chapter 1

Your Essence

There is a river of joy that is flowing inside of you.
Find it, go there, get in, and drown.

— Paramahansa Yogananda

For a while I had a podcast called "Stop Suffering About," where I interviewed those teachers and coaches who are exploring the understanding I'm sharing in this book. Each of the interviews was amazing in its own way, and I loved doing the show. And there was one particular moment from the 22 episodes that I did that really stood out to me among many, many amazing moments.

I was interviewing Anna Debenham, who created and runs an organization called the Insight Alliance. Their staff and volunteers work in prisons, bringing this understanding to prisoners with the aim of transforming their lives and ending recidivism. We talked about her work and how and why she got started, and then I asked her, "Where do you even begin when you're working with prisoners?"

My question came from the sense that when we're talking about well-being and the peace and wisdom that are innate to everyone, how do you introduce that to a group of people who may be spending the rest of their lives locked in a cage? People who have possibly grown up in the harshest, cruelest of circumstances, who may not ever have had a kind word spoken to them?

Anna explained that she begins by introducing the idea of our innate well-being. She asks the participants in her program to close their eyes and think of a moment when they felt a sense of peace or felt simply okay. Then she asks them to share what the qualities of that feeling were, and she writes the words the participants share on a whiteboard or flipchart. Calm, they say. Connected. Hope. Love. Understanding.

Then she asks, "What did you do to create that feeling?" The answer, over and over, is that they did nothing. It just happens, and the feeling is there. In other words, the participants didn't manufacture those feelings, those qualities of well-being; they simply exist and are present.

Anna points out that these feelings are not something we have to learn. And they are not something that is only available to certain people. This feeling, this calm, peace, love—whatever you want to call it—is built into each and every person. It is factory installed. And more than that, it's not just *part* of who we are: it *is* who we are. Those qualities are the materials that we are constructed from.

This innate well-being, this resilience we all share, never goes away. So, a person might have murdered someone (and some of those Anna works with have literally done that), but they too are always and forever built of well-being and resilience.

I was listening intently, interested in what she had to say. "Isn't this lovely?" I thought. I felt I understood what she was pointing to. I had been learning about this understanding for a couple of years at that point.

Then, Anna really blew my mind.

She went on to say that she'd recently had a prisoner react to this exercise with defiance. He said he'd never felt the feelings his fellow inmates were describing. He didn't have one instance of feeling even simply okay. He grew up in terrible circumstances and he'd had to fight his whole life, he explained. Anna asked him more about the fighting, and he described it. Then she asked, "Can you count on it?"

Yes, the participant said. He could always count on it, on the ability to fight and defend himself. He had done it his whole life.

Anna pointed out that this, too, is resilience. It is well-being. It may not look like peace and love, but it's the same. It points to a person's innate ability to take care of themselves, to protect themselves, to ensure they are safe.

That's well-being.

And this was when I grasped this understanding at a much deeper level: Every single person who has ever lived is made of this same resilience.

Including you.

Chapter 2

Week Two

That first Weight Watchers meeting was slightly intimidating, not least because they had us weigh in. Once our group was in the meeting room, we lined up in an orderly queue and, one‑by‑one, took our shoes off and stepped up onto a scale. I seem to recall the scale was the doctor's type, with the little weights that you slide along an arm until the arm balances. The woman weighing us jotted my number down on my weight tracking card—we'd all been given one—and handed it back to me. After that, the meeting progressed with motivational talks and explanations about the Weight Watchers system of the time. This was in the days before smart phones, so I vaguely recall that the system was about writing down what we'd eaten every day and tracking that using the points system assigned to various foods in a booklet we were given.

So far, so humiliating.

But it was the next week that things got really gnarly.

I arrived at the Sheraton again with an optimistic glow about me. I felt I'd had a pretty successful week tracking my food intake. I had certainly experienced the strain of trying to cut out some of my favorite comfort foods. At the time I was a sugar fiend. The only reason I ate a main course was so that I would feel justified having dessert. I was honest with myself that I had experienced some challenges cutting out the cake and cookie habit. But I had also been experiencing that temporary high that comes at the beginning of any new weight loss or self-improvement project. I could do this! It wasn't even that hard tracking what I was eating. I was a new woman and would soon have myself and my sugar addiction under control. You betcha!

Once again, we all lined up in the meeting room, like the polite Canadian ladies we were. Once again, as each person was weighed, the woman weighing us wrote their weight down on their card and handed it back to them. That week it was a bottle blonde with her hair cut in a Princess Diana style and a tight smile that didn't reach her eyes. Despite this, I noticed she was encouraging with everyone in the line in front of me.

"Great job, Donna! You're down half a pound."
"You lost another pound, Sally. Congratulations."
"Almost at your goal weight, Patricia. Well done!"

When it was my turn, I stepped up onto the scale and exchanged pleasantries with Princess Di. She moved the little weights back and forth across the arms of the scale.

Then she went quiet. She bent over and placed my card on the table beside her, picked up her pen, and wrote down her findings. She straightened up and handed me the card.

"Next!" she said, looking away from me.

Where's my encouragement? I thought.

I stepped off the scale and looked down at the card.

I'd gained a pound.

Chapter 3

You ARE Taking Care of Yourself

Your habit is a sign of your mental health.

— Dr. Amy Johnson

Fasten your seatbelt, because I'm about to turn your world upside down.

All of us assume, and all the diet gurus tell us, that overeating is self-sabotage. Or an 'addiction.' Or an absence of understanding that eating more than we need will lead to weight gain. (As if we can't do math.) We're doing harm to ourselves, they say, by eating too much and too often. So, we live with the shame of being overweight *and* the bonus guilt of believing ourselves to be people who are incapable of taking care of ourselves, not to mention lacking in basic math skills.

Worse, when we do try to 'take care of ourselves' by eating less or eating the 'right' foods, we inevitably fail. The message that we are somehow hell-bent to be unkind to ourselves is reinforced.

But what if those beliefs are all backward?

What if your drive to overeat is actually a sign of your innate health and well-being?

What if your 'bad habits' are your life's way of trying to get your attention and point out that you're caught up in a misunderstanding about who you are?

What are we doing when we reach for the cookie jar or the ice cream tub or the third donut? We're trying to soothe and comfort ourselves. In other words, we're trying to get in touch with feelings of calm and peace. Safety. Good feelings.

We've all felt it: that moment when we take the first bite of a 'forbidden' food or one we've been trying desperately to avoid. The feeling of relief that overtakes you. Perhaps an audible sigh escapes your lips. *Everything is going to be okay.*

This feeling might only last a second or two, until your brain starts to berate you about breaking your promise to not eat that thing. But for now, let's focus on how it feels when you decide to treat yourself, to indulge. Perhaps it feels like a matter of survival. You've had a really hard day and eating your special comfort food is going to fix that. And it absolutely does. You do feel better, even if it's momentarily.

Why is that?

Chapter 4

Being Human

Everyone is doing the best they can given the thinking they have that looks real to them.

— Sydney Banks

Before we go deeper into why this is happening to you specifically and why it's a sign of your mental health and well-being, let's pull our focus way back and look at humans in general for a moment.

Pretend you're visitng Earth from another planet and observing the human race as a scientist might. One thing you might notice right away is that habits and overindulgence exist everywhere, in all cultures and on all continents. Humans very often seem to refer to things they're 'addicted' to: food, alcohol, sex, drugs, shopping. This is not something that just a select group of humans experiences. Overindulgence, and the resulting shame, appear everywhere. They do not discriminate based on race, gender, locale, or the number of air miles a person has. And the humans you're observing seem to chalk this up to either filling an empty space within themselves, like they have a bottomless well to fill, or to a (misguided) attempt to fix something that is broken within them.

There are some humans who have everything they could possibly want. This is a smaller group, but they are interesting to observe because even when they have all the money, material goods, and security they could ever want, they can still struggle with the drive to overeat or over-drink or over-shop.

How can that be? It makes some sense that, if a human has very little or has a very stressful life, they would overindulge in order to feel better. But if someone has everything, shouldn't that drive to overindulge go away? This is very curious.

What you observe is that humans prefer to feel good. No one wants to be miserable. As an impartial observer, you can see that when humans do feel miserable, very simply, this is what that overindulgent behavior is trying to adjust and correct. They want to feel better. There is a universal drive to connect with a good feeling. Even for those who have everything.

Just like the need for food and shelter, the need to experience a feeling of peace is universal among humans, even when they don't realize that's what they're searching for.

There is an essence to every person, including you, that is more than your experiences, more than your knowledge, more than your personality and your preferences for disco over polka. This is what Anna Debenham is pointing toward in her work with prisoners when she shows them that good feelings—love, peace, calm—are not something we have to create. They're already there within us. They exist before and after us, outside the day-to-day events of our lives.

There is something beyond our human form that we are all made of. If we were all just a collection of flesh and bones and whirling atoms, would each and every one of us be able to describe this common experience of a good feeling? Would we be able to articulate the experience of searching for it, even if we weren't consciously aware of it?

Connecting to the feeling of well-being that we innately *are* will always override rules and willpower.

It has to.

The way being human works is that our drive to overeat is constantly reminding us who we are at our essence. It's not a mistake that you feel the drive to overeat. It's a reminder of your innate nature as a whole, and well, being.

This is why people experience habit switching. They stop smoking only to gain 25 pounds. Or they stop drinking but start smoking. Like a toddler that needs her mother's attention, your true nature of peace and well-being will not ever give up asking for you to notice it.

And here's the really amazing thing that absolutely blows my mind: when we widen our lens again, and look at what's common to all humans, we see that our innate but also *unconscious* awareness that peace and calm are our birthright is what, paradoxically, causes many of our 'problems.' The universal nature of what we call addictions proves this.

We are always trying to feel better, to connect with that which we instinctively know we really are.

And yes, it causes us to overeat.

It's like a game life plays with us. Hiding who we are from ourselves.

But if you pay attention, you'll see that nearly all the spiritual practices and teachings are pointing toward the same thing: your wholeness.

The drive to overeat is a gift. We think of it as a curse, but it's actually a very natural response to our true nature. We *are* well-being. It's just that sometimes we forget and need to be reminded.

Chapter 5

Dr. Phil

The secret is that you are already a completely whole, perfect person.

— Mavis Karn

I remember seeing an episode of the *Dr. Phil* show years ago, where he was talking to a woman who was dealing with the drive to overeat. This may have been in the era when his weight loss book had just been published.

When he was talking to this person about changing her habits, he recommended not having tempting foods in the house. I remember him saying something like, "If it's not in the house you're not going to go out and get it." He made it sound like this was so obvious. There was a 'duh' quality to his tone of voice.

Oh, dude, I thought, y*ou have no idea what you're talking about.*

OF COURSE we'll go out and get the food we want if it's not in our home. Someone who experiences the drive to overeat will walk barefoot through a snow storm in their pajamas to the corner store to buy that donut they so desperately need. Just try stopping them.

There's no shame in this. There's nothing wrong with that pajama-clad person. In fact, there is everything *right* with her.

The very nature of the drive that sends us to the fridge or the corner store when we know, logically, we don't want to be eating that fourth piece of cake or fifth donut —the *power* in that drive points to our wellness, not our brokenness or our lack of willpower.

We are using whatever means are available to us in the moment to feel the feeling of peace that is innately who we are. And if a donut is going to (temporarily) be a substitute for that feeling, then woe betide the person who gets in between us and that glorious glazed pastry.

Restricting ourselves from eating our favorite foods cuts us off from the simulated feelings of peace and wholeness that those foods give us. (Key word: simulated.) We are already unaware of our innate and true nature, our intrinsic peace and well-being; this causes us suffering, so when we try to refrain from eating the foods that simulate that true nature, it's just too much to cope with.

Sadly, we don't know this. As a result, we shame ourselves for behavior that is entirely natural. Without knowing there's an alternative way of seeing what's happening, we add layers of self-judgment to the negative thinking we already have about our habit.

Innocently, when Dr. Phil was inviting his guest to clear out her kitchen cupboards he was applying a strategy that seems logical. However, what that guest really needed was to be pointed toward her innate health and well-being. The contents of our cupboards isn't the problem. The problem is an innocent lack of awareness about the beauty, kindness, and divine perfection in our human design.

Chapter 6

The Self-Help Paradox

Your thoughts and feelings are a mirror of your soul.

— Sydney Banks

Have you got a PhD in self-help? Have you read dozens of books and invested way more than dozens of dollars to 'fix' yourself, to try and stamp out the drive to overeat?

Me too.

For those of us who are naturally introspective and interested in our own growth and healing, self-help makes sense. The generations before us didn't have the luxury of introspection or the information available to them that we have now. Self-help, as we know it today, didn't really start until the 1970s. There were a few books available earlier than this that we would now consider to be self-help books, like Napoleon Hill's *Think and Grow Rich*. But it was in the 70s that the movement really took off.

I became an adult in the 1990s and spent the next 30+ years devouring every self-help book I could find, taking classes and going to therapy, all with the aim of 'fixing' myself. Perhaps you've had a similar experience.

In hindsight, all that self-help work I did meant that I became highly attuned to my 'problems.' I can spot a psychological hitch in my giddy-up from miles away. We know all the lingo. We've practiced the affirmations. We've (probably) done the exercises in the workbooks.

I remember one particular weight loss program I enrolled in that, at the time, was called The Solution. The course cost a couple thousand dollars, I seem to recall, and I was shipped a set of six or seven weighty manuals. They were textbook sized; thick and intimidating. The course involved weekly telephone classes (this was before online video classes became the norm) and a metric ton of practicing and homework. On top of that studying, along with a group of five or six others in the class, I organized a telephone study group which met once a week. There was also an exercise-/mantra-type thing that we were taught, and I practiced that several times an hour. Every hour. For months.

Additionally, for the year I was taking that training, I blocked off every Sunday to work on the course materials. I did nothing else for that year of Sundays but sit on my couch and work my way through those manuals and faithfully do the exercises within. They were designed to excavate buried or suppressed emotions, so I dug deep, holding nothing back and writing in my journal until my fingers ached. I was *determined* that the money I'd invested in that course would not go to waste and that I'd be able to heal my food addiction.

Spoiler alert: It didn't work.

By the time the course was over, I was left feeling like there must be something really big that was wrong with me because the course had made little, if any, impact on my eating habits. Did that stop me from trying the next self-help program I found? No. Did it stop me from haunting the weight loss section of Vancouver's meta-physical bookstore? No again.

I'd bet good money you can relate to this story and probably have one (or more) of your own.

Those of us who are introspective and who have a natural bent toward wanting to do better and improve our lives know how to *work* at that. We are dogged— relentless, really—when it comes to wanting to find peace within ourselves. And as I mentioned previously, there's a perfectly natural and healthy reason for that: we have a natural drive to connect with our innate sense of peace.

However, what often happens is that drive to find peace takes us down the wrong road: it may create a habit of working really hard and looking diligently at the 'problems' we have, rather than helping us turn our attention toward unearthing the peace and well-being that is innate within us and always available to us.

The illustration below shows how the old self-help paradigm works.

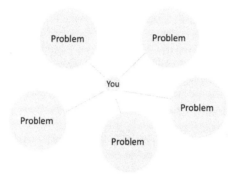

In this old self-help paradigm, our focus is, innocently, on the problems we perceive that we have. Makes sense, right? If you've got a burned-out light bulb or a plugged toilet, focusing on those problems and working on them is what fixes them. So, if I feel there's something wrong with me, then my best approach is to focus on that problem and try to fix it. This is only logical.

Additionally, my experience was that the more educated I became about personal growth and traditional (old paradigm) psychology, the more problems I could see in myself. My awareness of what was 'wrong' with me only made me more attuned to other issues I could poten-tially have.

There's an expression I love that says, 'If the only tool you have is a hammer, then everything looks like a nail.' In the context of this chapter, if the only tool you have is the old paradigm of self-help, then everything we think and feel can look like a problem that needs to be fixed.

In the last few decades, it has become much more widely accepted, at least in Western culture, to talk about our 'issues' and how we're going to therapy to work on ourselves. We're all more educated about our feelings and about the language around human psychology. And, in a way, this is great. It's certainly better than being emotionally shut down and repressed. But at the same time, when we're almost entirely focused on our perceived brokenness, we're looking in the wrong direction.

The inside-out understanding points us in a different direction.

You =
Wisdom / Serenity
/ Insight / Well-
being / Resilience

This is a new paradigm of wholeness, rather than brokenness. Each of us, every human who has ever existed, is whole and well at our essence. We are incorruptible and have infinite access to resourcefulness, peace, and well-being. Even when we are ill or incarcerated or financially broke, the essence of who we are never changes.

When we stop thinking of ourselves as a conglomeration of wounds and problems stitched together like a quilt made of discarded pieces of clothing and instead turn toward our innate well-being, those problems we perceived begin to have less significance.

Healing the drive to overeat isn't about finding all the things you believe are wrong with you and fixing them. It's about coming to understand that there's nothing wrong with you in the first place.

Chapter 7

The Sky

Whatever has the nature to arise, will also pass away.

— The Buddha

The old paradigm of psychology, the one most of us are used to and have absorbed unconsciously via cultural language and norms, says that we are born whole and perfect and then gradually over time become 'damaged' and worn down by life, like a worn-out running shoe or a bald set of car tires. Life, we believe, has an impact on us; it can bend and break us with its painful experiences and traumatic events.

We've all had hard times, or worse, and we've all experienced loss and heartbreak and perhaps even trauma. Challenging upbringings bereft of affection, or maybe just lacking the kind of affection we wanted. Car accidents. Disease. Disappointments that are small or some-times profound. Life happens to everyone. No one is exempt from the multitudinous, varied, and often really daunting experiences of being human.

And we often carry these experiences around with us each day, if not physically in the form of injuries, then mentally in the form of anger, resentment, fear, sadness, or hurt feelings.

A human being is a small creature in a vast world full of the potential for scraped knees, flooded basements, and expensive, not to mention sad, divorces.

But what if you are more than a meat popsicle being slowly chomped by your life experiences?

What if you are more like the sky—a vast and infinite space that weather simply moves through?

The weather, no matter how dramatic and dangerous-looking, has zero effect on the sky. Even when your view of the sky is entirely blotted out by black clouds, light-ning, and sheets of rain, the blue sky is still there; it is just momentarily obscured. Weather moves *through* the sky; it does not have an impact on it. Ever. In the millions of years the Earth has been in existence, the fiercest of storms has never had a single, minute effect on the sky.

You are the sky.

You have experiences in life, and, yes, some of them are really hard and awful, but no matter their content those experiences can never affect your true nature, your vast and immutable fabric.

We see this everywhere. We see it in children who are raised in neglectful and unloving homes who not only go on to achieve great things, but perhaps even more importantly, are able to offer love and compassion to others. We see it in those who are physically injured in some way but who continue to approach life with joy and an open heart. We see poets, filmmakers, and other artists point toward this truth in works of art that move us to tears when we recognize in them the resilience, connection, love, and kindness that surround us and that are the very fabric of our own cells. We read it in the poetry written by inmates during incarceration. We hear it in gospel songs that lift the heart.

I'm going to come back to this metaphor and explore its deeper layers later, but for now, I just want to plant the seed. What if you are more than you think you are?

Part Two

The River of Life

Chapter 8

Changing Schools

You are not a problem.

— Mavis Karn

By the time my 50th year on planet Earth rolled around, I'd been battling with my overeating habit for 30 years. I was bloodied, bruised, and humiliated, but I kept going. In fact, I had been on my quest for so long, I realized I'd started to circle back around to many of the strategies that had failed me in the past. For example, after my disastrous experience with Weight Watchers in the early 90s, I'd signed up for it again at least twice. I'd also re-explored other methods I'd tried in the past that hadn't worked, thinking I must have missed something, or hadn't explored the strategy deeply enough or spent enough time on it.

In other words, I believed that the failures and flaws lay within me, not with the strategies themselves, so I kept giving them another try. Tragically, I failed again, and again, and again, and, what's worse, the conclusion I came to after all that failure was that *I* was the problem. I began to believe that something must be deeply and inherently wrong with me, given that all the help in the world, and all the focus and effort I'd put in, weren't able to fix my overeating habit.

What a terrible feeling. I carried the shame of it around with me everywhere I went. I hated shopping for clothes because almost everything cute that I wanted to wear didn't come in my size. I put off doing things I wanted to do—like learn to kayak—until I lost weight. I wasn't living my life; I was just existing until some undetermined moment in the future when I'd fixed the dreadful thing about me.

What I wish I had seen then is that I wasn't the problem at all; I know this now. I recently heard a metaphor that made me think of myself and those 30 years of 'failure': if you judge a fish for its ability climb a tree it's going to live its whole life believing it's stupid.

I believed that when it came to eating reasonably and not feeling the compulsive drive to eat too much, I was stupid. That I was somehow not grasping what the weight loss industry was trying to tell me.

I couldn't have been more wrong about that.

I wasn't stupid. Or broken. I was simply a student seeking knowledge in the wrong school. I valiantly tried all sorts of different classrooms, but behind every door I knocked on was the same information, just worded differently.

Thankfully, in the summer I turned 50 a friend introduced me to the understanding I'm sharing in this book. At first, I was baffled by it. I started following several practitioners in this field and noticed that the style of teaching and sharing information was less about offering concrete, step-by-step solutions (i.e., do this, then do that —the model I was familiar with, even if it didn't work), and more about describing what they saw to be true about our human experience. But gradually, as I listened and read more, it began to make sense to me.

Sometimes, in order to get the results we're looking for, we have to change schools entirely.

Chapter 9

Let's Fly a Kite

A woman, let's call her Alice, is driving to work one day. It is a blustery, windy day, and as she drives down her street, she sees her neighbor running around her driveway in a strange, jerky way. As Alice approaches, she sees that her neighbor's garbage can has been knocked over and pieces of paper and plastic are being whirled about. The neighbor is trying to catch them, collect them, and put them back in the garbage can. Her face is grim and unhappy. Alice stops the car, gets out, and helps wrangle the flying litter back into the garbage can.

"What a disaster," the neighbor says, as they put the lid on the can. "Now my whole day is ruined."

Alice gets back in her car and continues her journey, and when she reaches the end of the block, she passes the large, green park that is the feature of her neighborhood. A family is flying kites, which being lifted, effortlessly, up into the air by the strong breezes. Alice notices the smiles of delight on the family's faces. Even their dog is running happily with them, joining in on the fun.

Two very different experiences, Alice thinks, but it's the same wind.

Chapter 10

Inside-Out

We live in the world of our thinking, not in the world of our experiences.

— Michael Neill

I'm going to lay out two scenarios for you.

In the first, you are in a very peaceful setting, perhaps reading a book on a beach. The situation around you is calm and quiet. There are no crowds or noise, just the sound of the waves lapping at the shore and maybe the occasional call of a sea bird.

In the second, you are in a busy office setting and the printer you use to print out the reports for a Very Important Client who is arriving in 10 minutes has just broken down.

Now, in scenario A (the beach), how do you imagine you'd be feeling? What about in scenario B (the office)?

For scenario A, you might think you'd be feeling calm, quiet, relaxed. And for scenario B you might imagine being anxious or stressed.

But let's take a step back for a second. What if in scenario A you're someone who is easily bored and prefers vacations that involve adventure, exploration, and learning new things? And what if in scenario B you are someone who has worked toward your current job for a decade and thrived on the challenge and excitement that the job presents?

Or we can look at it another way. What if in scenario A you'd just had a memory of a fight you had with a friend six months ago? And what if in scenario B your hands are busy doing a task but your mind is remembering your beautiful new baby niece (or something else with a lovely feeling attached to it)?

We've all been in a situation where we expected to be happy and content, yet didn't actually feel that way. Maybe it was something similar to the beach vacation I describe above. All the right pieces are in place, and maybe you'd been looking forward to that experience for months, but when you get there, you don't feel calm or happy or even content.

When we take a step back and look at our thinking with a slightly objective eye, we can see that we are not having thoughts because of our outside circumstances. Our thinking is actually coming to life from within us. At any moment, in any given circumstance, we can have any type of thought. Happy thoughts in challenging times and dark thoughts in happy times.

When we believe that our thinking is caused by the things happening outside ourselves (outside-in), we give the credit for a busy or a quiet mind to those circumstances. If someone is reading a book on a beach, then their thinking is likely calm and quiet. If that same person is juggling a number of complicated tasks in a busy office setting, then their mind is likely stirred up.

Makes sense, right?

Except that when we consider this assumption, we can likely see that in our own lives there are times when this is not true. We can be on that beach on our dream vacation, with the waves gently lapping at the shore and the occasional cry of a seagull overhead, and our thoughts can be a whirling dervish of fear or anger or anxiety. There can be nothing in front of us but sand and surf and sunshine, and we can be as miserable or angry or fraught as we have ever been.

And the opposite is true as well. It's possible you've had the experience of being in a situation where you had anticipated you'd be feeling anxious or upset, only to realize you feel happy or calm.

Our thinking is energy, coming to life within us, moment to moment. And we live in the world of that thinking, not in the world of what's happening outside ourselves.

When we first encounter this idea, it can seem absurd, but bear with me and we'll explore why it's so important when it comes to ending the drive to overeat.

Chapter 11

Email

Tension reminds me I already have what I'm looking for.

— Dicken Bettinger

In the early aughts, my mother was living in Bolivia for a few months with her husband, my stepfather. He was teaching pipeline engineers about North American practices, and my mom had joined him to experience life in another country.

We exchanged emails regularly, and she shared lots of interesting anecdotes about the culture, customs, and food, among other things, and about the adventures they were having.

One day I received an email from her and sat reading it at my desk. Something she said sent me into a fury. (I can't remember what it was now.) I was enraged in a way I rarely am. I recall pacing around my home office, mentally composing the response that I would send to her incredibly offensive and hurtful email. I will be articulate but cutting, I told myself. I will skillfully and artfully use the power of words to tell her why and how she was so profoundly wrong and how deeply she has hurt me.

I sat down to write my reply and, in a brief but profound moment of clarity, I realized I was too angry to write the letter. I decided I should wait, possibly overnight, and then approach the problem with fresh eyes.

So that's what I did. I didn't look at her email for the rest of the day. My mind was still stirred up, but gradually I was distracted by work and life and forgot about it momentarily.

The next morning, the first thing on my agenda was to compose my *magnum opus* email, letting my mother know exactly what was what. To refresh my memory, I opened her email and reread what she said. As I read, I saw that there was one word that my eyes had skipped over when I'd read the email the day before. And I realized that this word changed the entire context of what she'd said.

Suddenly my whole world shifted. My rage and self-righteousness collapsed.

There was nothing to be angry at. Absolutely nothing. She hadn't said or meant what I thought. The whole episode of having been so angry I couldn't sit still had been entirely made up in my head.

We experience life from the inside-out, not the other way around.

My angry and self-righteous response was not to my mother's email; it was to my thoughts about her email.

We live in the world of our thinking, not in the world of our experiences.

Chapter 12

The Sky, Part 2

Every storm runs out of rain.

— Maya Angelou

For part of my growing up, I lived in southern Alberta. There's a popular saying there that if you don't like the weather, wait five minutes. This is just one of the funnier ways of addressing the changeable and temporary nature of the weather in that part of the world. I've since heard that expression in other places, which makes sense, because the weather is changeable wherever we go.

This brings us back to our sky metaphor from a few chapters ago.

Just like the weather outside your window, the 'weather' inside you is always changing, and it does so on its own.

Moving and flowing like the clouds through the sky. And just like those clouds, our thoughts and feelings are largely out of our control. They come and go on their own, sometimes stormy, sometimes calm. And behind that moveable, changeable weather is the blue sky. Never changing. Always there, even when we can't see it. This blue sky is our true nature that doesn't change: peace, well-being, resilience.

In a previous section, I described the scenario of being on a dream vacation. If we *could* control our thoughts and feelings, wouldn't everyone who was on a dream vacation be thinking happy thoughts and feeling happy feelings for the duration of that vacation? Of course. And yet, every day, people on dream vacations have thoughts and feelings that range from the mundane to the dramatic, and back again.

We live with an innocent misunderstanding that we can control, or even just have an effect on, our thoughts and feelings. This misunderstanding is what leads us to develop our overeating habit.

We innocently believe that eating something (or drinking something or smoking something) gives us control over the weather inside us. Metaphorically, we use food to try to connect ourselves to our blue sky.

The beauty of this is that once we begin to see the changeable nature of the weather within us and how it comes and goes on its own—and that we aren't responsible for it, and it isn't personal—our need to control the weather with food drops away all on its own. Once we understand that every storm does indeed run out of rain, our innocent drive to try to control the storm begins to look absurd.

Chapter 13

Soda Story, Part 1

I was standing in my local grocery store, bent over at the waist, with what must have been a very strange look on my face. I was all at once puzzled, thrilled, and marveling at the miraculous nature of my body and my being.

Let me back up and explain.

For close to 30 years, I had a daily Coke habit. Not the powdered kind that gets sniffed up the nose, but the liquid kind that comes in a can or bottle. I don't know exactly when it started, but I do remember being in my early 20s, working at a summer job for a natural gas company in the records department, and finding myself going to the vending machine every day at lunch. Even then, in the very early days of feeling the drive to overeat, I was uncomfortable having a soda every day at lunch. It was always just one, I said to myself, justifying. But still, I didn't think it was very healthy and I didn't like the feeling of need attached to it.

Over the next 30 years, quitting this habit became my version of smoking. It was easy to quit, as the joke goes; it was just that I started up again the next day, or two days later at most. This daily habit gradually became a millstone around my neck. By the time I got to my early 30s I was really embarrassed by it. And ashamed. What kind of adult drinks sugary soda every day? I kept trying to quit and kept failing.

And the habit puzzled me with its specificity and characteristics. It had to be the Coca-Cola brand, never any other kind. It was always the full sugar version, never diet. It had to be in a can, never a plastic bottle. (I thought it tasted better from the metal can.) And there were times when, even if I'd been out to lunch with work colleagues and had had fountain soda with my meal, I'd still feel driven to have a can of Coke when I got back to my desk. It was like a comfort blanket or a soother that a toddler needs. Gut instinct told me I was minimally addicted to the sugar and caffeine, and mostly addicted to the perceived comfort I derived from the habit.

I kept trying to quit and kept failing all through my 30s and 40s. I'd try strategies like switching to carbonated water but, as ever, that only worked for a day or two. And this habit was on my mind a *lot*. I felt like it was a visible signal to the world, a big sign over my head saying, "This person has a drive-to-overeat problem. She's a loser."

Not fun.

Then in mid-2017, as I've mentioned, I started to learn about this inside-out understanding. Early on in my learning, as I began to learn the things I'm sharing in this book, I eased up on beating myself up about my habits. This was a relief, even though they persisted, including my soda habit.

At some point, I don't remember exactly when, I noticed that when I sat down for lunch every day with my can of Coke, I would drink less than a third of it and then pour the rest down the sink after I finished eating my lunch. So I switched to buying the mini-cans that, at 222 mL or about 8 ounces, are a little more than half the size of the regular 355 mL / 12-oz. size. (I live in Canada so we measure liquids in milliliters rather than ounces.) This seemed like a step in the right direction in terms of letting go of this habit, and I was pleased.

A while later—again, I'm not sure how long—was when I found myself in the grocery store with the strange look on my face.

I had been walking up and down the aisles, as you do, putting items into my little red basket and checking the grocery list on my phone. My last stop was the soda, chip, and bottled water aisle. I walked over to where the cans of Coke were, bent over toward the shelf where they were housed, and was reaching for a six-pack of the mini-cans when my whole body went, "Meh."

That 'meh' told me that my body was entirely uninterested in buying those little cans of soda. Hence my expression of stunned puzzlement and wonder.

It took me a few seconds to realize that I was frozen, my arm outstretched, feeling that 'meh' feeling and being both dazzled and confused by it. There were other people in the aisle, so I straightened up and stepped out of the way in order to check in with myself about what was going on. I stood off to the side and pictured myself reaching for the mini-cans and putting them in my basket. My previously beloved lunch drink, the magical elixir that had been my constant companion (and nemesis) for 30 years. My daily 'fix' of comfort and routine and sugary goodness.

"Meh," my body said again.

So I exited the aisle. I went to the front of the store, paid for my groceries and left *sans* mini-cans. I walked home in a state of wonder, knowing immediately and emphatically that this extraordinary event was due to my exploration of the inside-out understanding. I had 30 years of empirical evidence of trying to force myself to stop a habit and failing miserably. And here I was, *not* forcing myself to stop anything, and yet this deeply ingrained habit had just fallen away, without any willpower or mental machinations on my part.

Astounding.

And to my amazement, the revelation continued: my lunch the next day was even more interesting, and I experienced for myself one of the most important ideas behind this understanding. More on that in a minute.

Chapter 14

River of Life

Thought is not reality. However, our personal realities are molded through our thoughts.

— Sydney Banks

In the introduction to Amanda Jones' book *Uncovery*, Dr. Amy Johnson introduces the idea that our thinking is like a river. Not only is our thinking coming from the inside out, it is flowing energy, always moving, always changing, just like the clouds in the sky we talked about in a previous chapter.

We humans are a part of nature, so comparing the energy of thought to the natural form of a moving body of water makes perfect sense. When we look at nature, we can see that it is so often in motion. The obvious examples are oceans and rivers. But even when we look at slightly different examples, we see motion. The way any animal, human or otherwise, is constantly changing; growing from a baby into an adult and then aging until death, shedding cells that are constantly being replaced, growing hair and nails continually, digesting food and expelling it.

I love watching the flowers that I plant on my balcony for this reason. They are never the same from one day to the next, always growing and moving. And then, when the days grow shorter and the air becomes chill, the annuals that I planted wither and die, after which they go into the compost, where they continue to change, decaying and transforming into something that will provide life for other plants and animals.

Even mountains are in motion, either being thrust higher into the sky by the movement of the Earth's plates, or being eroded by the rain and wind that batter them.

Nature is movement. And we are a part of nature. As is our thinking.

Our thinking is a river of thought that is coming to life within us, moment to moment (as Dr. Amy says), never the same from one moment to the next. Sometimes this river is calm and quiet, trickling along, playing music over the rocks and pebbles in its bed. Other times, it is raging, water surging and breaking in frothy, wild torrents.

But no matter what the 'mood' of that river of thoughts is, it is always moving. You can count on that 100 percent. Don't quite believe me? Just try to hold one thought in your mind for the next 10 minutes. If you've ever meditated, you'll know how impossible that is.

This continual, eternal movement is a gift because it means we don't have to hang on to or make meaning of any one thought in any given moment. Another thought, perhaps a gentler, kinder thought, will be along in the next moment. And the next.

In the introduction to Amanda's book, Dr. Amy likens our propensity for getting attached to our thoughts to taking a bucket and going to that river that flows through us, dipping the bucket in the river and then walking around all day holding onto that bucket. If we're lucky, the water in the bucket is clear. But often that is not the case. The buckets of water we sometimes hold on to are full of sticks and mud and leaves and other detritus.

When we see that our thinking changes from moment to moment, that it moves and flows, and that this is true for all humans everywhere, then we understand that we don't have to be attached to any one thought in any given moment.

Alternatively, what you and I have been doing—innocently—when we have a thought about eating a second bowl of ice cream or a fifth cookie or having that fourth glass of wine is getting attached to that thought and carrying it around with us. Just like that bucket of water I talked about a minute ago.

"What does it say about me that I have that thought?" we ask ourselves. And we answer, "It means I'm weak willed. It means I'm sabotaging myself. It means I'm damaged and broken."

And then we're off to the races, wondering why we can't control ourselves and why the drive to overeat controls our lives.

When instead, all that's happened is that a leaf has floated down the river. And when we stand on the bank and notice that leaf, we can watch it go by without making it mean anything. Without having to dip our bucket in and pull the leaf out and carry it around in the bucket. It's just a leaf. In a moment another one might float by. Or a stick. Or a fish. Or a rubber inner tube.

None of those things means anything about who you are.

Chapter 15

Your Innate Superpower

Feelings exist to warn us away from using our thinking to create trouble in our lives and to guide us back to our natural, healthy ability to live our lives to the fullest.

— Mavis Karn

L ife is wise. It knows how to put the plants to sleep in the fall and wake them back up in the spring. It knows that sunrise follows sunset. It guides baby ducklings to follow their mama. It works in the leaves of trees to turn carbon dioxide and water into oxygen. It knows how to knit bones when they're broken.

Life has also designed a perfect feedback system within you that lets you know when you're caught up in thinking that isn't peaceful, loving, and healthy: thinking that isn't coming from your resilient, wise nature. That system is your feelings. And this is your innate superpower.

The sensations in our body are a perfect feedback system to show us what we're thinking and *that* we're thinking.

The story I told earlier about receiving an email from my mom and reacting to something she hadn't said is a perfect illustration of this. All those feelings of anger and self-righteousness, all that churning in my stomach, fizzing in my head, and tightness in my chest was life's way of holding up a flag to get my attention. "You're caught up in your thinking. You're living with a misunderstanding at the moment."

It is our nature to be peaceful, joyful, fully alive, happy, loving, and optimistic. When we stray away from this, our feelings are there—the perfect feedback system—to let us know what has happened.

This system is perfect because it always, always alerts us when we're caught up in thinking that doesn't serve us. It is never asleep on the job.

Paradoxically, and innocently, we often interpret our feelings to mean something about us or about the situation we're in. "I felt anxious driving over that bridge; therefore, bridges must be dangerous and I should avoid them in future." Or, "I'm irritated with my spouse about how he loads the dishwasher; therefore, he needs to change or I won't be happy and my life will be ruined."

The feelings within us that I call the drive to overeat are saying, "Hey, no judgment here, but you're caught up in thinking that you need to manage and control the clouds in the sky." When we see that feeling—the drive—for what it is, it becomes less 'sticky' and gradually begins to fade away altogether.

Chapter 16

The Lead Mare

It is early autumn 2014 and I'm standing in a covered outdoor riding arena. Beyond the open walls I can see the California sunshine warming the desert landscape. Here inside, it's a bit chilly in the early morning, and I'm wishing I'd worn a light jacket.

The arena is huge, probably nearly the length of a football field and almost as wide. The ground is covered in brown dirt, and where the sun comes past the walls into the building, I can see dust motes floating in the beams. Within the larger arena, there's a temporary round pen that's about 40 feet in diameter. I'm inside that pen and I'm not alone. With me is a brown and white horse, whose name I didn't catch, and we're going to spend the next few minutes bonding.

I'm here at 'horsey camp,' as I call it, in my latest attempt to try to heal the drive to overeat. I've flown from Vancouver, British Columbia, to very Southern

California and spent money I don't have in order to spend two days doing what's called Equus training.

I love horses and grew up around them. My dad started me taking riding lessons when I was about four years old. So this is a comfortable and happy place for me. However, we're not doing any riding this weekend. I and the other ten or so women in the class will all be doing our work from the ground. Which is why I'm standing in the round pen with a paint horse.

Over the next two days, we all take turns in the round pen with a variety of horses. The premise of the training is that we're going to learn about ourselves by being in the pen with a horse, both by seeing how we react to different situations and also by seeing how the horses react to us. Horses are highly intuitive and sensitive crea-tures. Though they are large, they are prey animals, not predators, so they've evolved to be keenly sensitive to their environments and to changes in the energy around them. As such, they give *immediate* feedback about a person's state of being, often pointing out patterns of behavior that we aren't aware of.

The objective of the first exercise we do is to get the horse to trot, or canter, around the outside edge of the round pen. Individual trainees like me stand in the very center of the pen and encourage the horse to move without shouting or running at it. You might have a coiled lead rope in one hand that you can gently slap against your leg, but that's all the guidance you can give to the large animal looking at you with wary eyes. You're essentially moving the horse with your energy. Letting it know what you want it to do by holding the intention in your mind and being clear and calm. (We'll get to why calmness matters in a minute.)

I've traveled to this foreign land, crossed an international boundary, rented a car, and booked a hotel with the hope that this silent, brown and white animal with pointy ears and a soft muzzle will show me what's wrong with me. I want to know why I feel so broken inside and why, no matter what I do, I can't seem to conquer the drive to overeat.

The horse and I look at one another for a few moments while I receive instruction from the workshop trainer. Outside the round pen, my fellow workshop participants are watching, which is really uncomfortable for me. I hate being the center of attention.

The workshop leader, Jill (not her real name), lets me know I can start anytime. I picture in my mind what I want to happen, gently flap the lead rope against my jeans, and make a clucking sound with my tongue. The horse starts to move, trotting counterclockwise around the pen.

After a few moments, Jill says, "Get her to canter," so I hold that intention in my mind and, miraculously, the horse starts to canter.

I can feel the connection between me and the horse. My self-consciousness about being watched disappears and my attention is entirely focused on the present moment, here, in this round pen with this brown and white horse.

"Now make her turn around so she's going in the other direction," Jill says.

I keep my energy at the center of myself (I'm not sure how else to describe this), step ever so slightly to my left, and imagine the horse turning around and running in the other direction.

And it does.

I'm elated.

"Now slow her down."

I calm my energy down, sort of like pulling a blind down over a sunny window, and the horse slows down from its canter to a trot, then a walk.

"Excellent," Jill says. "How was that for you?"

I turn my back on the horse and look through the bars of the round pen at Jill and the others who are standing in the dirt outside it. I can hear the horse coming up behind me and eventually it comes to stand beside my right shoulder as I describe what the experience was like for me. I turn slightly and place my hand on the horse's withers while I speak. Someone in the group takes a photo of me and the paint horse, and to this day, I have that image pinned to my fridge.

As I said, I grew up around horses, but this experience was entirely different than saddling and unsaddling, walking, trotting, and cantering (heels down!), and jumping over little rails. There was more connection between me and that brown and white gelding in those 20 minutes than there had ever been with any of the horses I'd ridden as a child and teenager.

And yet, I leave the weekend disappointed.

I get to spend a couple more sessions in the round pen with different horses over the course of the weekend and each time it is as effortless and powerful as the first time. Others in the group have different experiences, and several have big, cathartic moments that are akin to a breakthrough in therapy, except they do it standing on a dirt floor and sobbing into the neck of a doe-eyed gelding or mare. I don't experience this. I don't come any closer to understanding why I feel the drive to overeat, and I leave the weekend grateful for the experience but very sad. I had wanted to be fixed. Surely spending all that money and traveling all that way would have resulted in some sort of healing awareness. But it didn't.

I do learn one thing, though, that sticks with me from then on, and it is this. Every wild horse herd has a lead mare. It is her responsibility to guide the herd to good grazing areas and to sources of water. She will also alert the herd to signs of danger. And the most interesting thing about a lead mare is that she is not necessarily the toughest animal in the herd; she's not necessarily the strongest, fastest, or biggest. She's the calmest.

Now, if you're an equine biologist you might dispute the veracity of this claim, but I love this as a metaphor. It points to the idea that being calm serves us.

This little nugget of information stays with me in the years leading away from that workshop, popping into my head every once in a while. And once I discover the inside-out understanding, I will see how it is a helpful metaphor for our human experience and for healing the drive to overeat.

Chapter 17

Snow Globe

What everyone is searching for is a quiet mind, and there lies the answer.

— Sydney Banks

Have you ever bought one of those kitschy snow globes from a tourist location? The kind that are about the side of a softball, or smaller, and have a flat bottom. They usually have a scene of some sort inside, a cityscape in miniature or an animal or a North Pole scene. When they're shaken up, 'snow' flies around inside the globe, temporarily suspended in the watery substance that fills it.

Your mind (and mine) is like that snow globe. It can get really shaken up and busy with thoughts swirling around. It can seem really stormy inside there at times, and it can feel as though the snowflakes will never stop swirling. And in response to this, we can develop strategies for dealing with those swirling thoughts; maybe an extra glass of wine to soothe ourselves, or picking a fight with a friend to distract ourselves and drown out the noise.

But here's the thing about snow globes and minds: if we leave them alone, they quiet down all by themselves. You don't have to do anything to make the flakes inside the snow globe stop swirling. If you leave the globe alone, the flakes settle down on their own.

We use lots of metaphors when we're talking about the inside-out understanding because they're such a powerful way to convey new ideas. This is one of my particular favorites and one that was really helpful to me when I was first learning about this understanding.

We humans are thinking creatures. We come to life equipped with enormous problem-solving brains. So, often, when we have a problem—say, for example, when we feel a drive to overeat—we can innocently add more thinking to that problem, assuming that this will help. But, perhaps counterintuitively, it is often when our minds are settled that the most helpful ideas come to us.

Adding more thinking to a problem is like shaking up that snow globe while expecting it to settle. But like the lead mare in the previous story, we are at our best, and most helpful to others, when we are calm. When we see that we don't need to do anything to create a state of calm—that the snow globe settles down all by itself—we can simply wait, and clarity will return.

When I was six or seven years old, I fell on an icy patch of snow and broke my right arm. When I got home (this was the 70s, so kids were free range) my mom took me to emergency and they put a cast on my arm.

A few years later, when my brother was about the same age, he ran headlong into a wooden banister and cut the top of his head open. His scalp bled like crazy and he had to get five or six stitches.

When we injure our bodies, we use the tools available to us to repair them: bandages, stitches, plaster casts, splints, and ointment.

And, innocently, when we misunderstand where our emotional experience is coming from, we do the same for our feelings.

Had a bad day? Put some alcohol on it (as the Brad Paisley song goes).

Furious with your spouse? Put a bowl of ice cream on it.

Sad about losing a job you loved? Stitch up that wound with a piece of chocolate cake.

The problem with this strategy, as innocent as it is, is that we are a river of feelings that is in perpetual motion. Our experience is coming to life, moment to moment, and there's no need to stitch it up with anything. It's not broken. In fact, it works perfectly well without our interference.

Our emotional body is self-correcting, just like that snow globe. When we leave our thoughts and feelings alone, they settle down on their own. Maybe not immediately, but 100 percent of the time they do change and settle.

I know with absolute certainty that the way I feel now is not the way I'll feel in the future. I could bet ten million dollars on that and I'd win every time.

My overeating habit formed when I had this understanding backward. When I thought that I needed to do something to feel better, I developed the habit of using food to do that.

Chapter 18

Family

My dad, who is 80 as I write this, texts me every day to tell me what he's having for lunch. He usually goes to an Italian restaurant and has his favorite meal: lamb shanks with vegetables. It's something he looks forward to every day, a tasty highlight in a quiet retirement life.

I come from a family that is riddled, on both sides, with what I used to describe as addictions. Overeating, overspending, overdrinking. And I used to have a lot of thinking about that. "How on earth can I expect to break free of my drive to overeat if addiction runs in my family? It's hereditary," I'd say to myself. "I'm doomed."

Turns out, that wasn't true. What's happening in a family like mine, where there is more than one person dealing with the drive toward 'over-ing,' is that we're all simply operating under the same innocent misunderstandings.

I was never doomed. My DNA is responsible for my hair and eye color, perhaps the shape of my legs or how easily I freckle in the sun. But my overeating habit is not tied to my family. And it's not tied to my tumultuous and sometimes neglectful upbringing, nor to the traumas I've experienced.

The more I turn my attention toward seeing what so many wise people have been pointing toward—that life is living through me, that I am whole and resilient, that there is not now, nor has there ever been, anything wrong with me—the more that snow globe in my mind settles and the more I am free of my overeating habit.

Chapter 19

Vertical Blinds

That's what a mind does.

— Dr. Amy Johnson

There is a window between you and your experiences. And the factory that installed that window also installed a set of vertical blinds.

Some days the blinds are pulled all the way to one side and you can see clearly, observing the bright blue sky outside and the sunshine as it lands on the flowers in your front yard. Other days the blinds are pulled across the window, blocking out some of your view. Sometimes they're turned so that they create a wall between you and the view. Other times they are set at an angle so that you can see part of the view, broken up into tall, rectangular sections.

Meanwhile, the world on the other side of the glass is simply going about its business. Life is life-ing.

The blinds represent our thoughts about that world and that life. Sometimes they obscure the view very little and we're able to observe what's happening without much thinking about it. Other times they block the view entirely and we can only see our thinking about a situation.

Most of the time, though, the blinds are somewhere in between and we have some thinking about the view.

The blinds, as I said, are factory installed. There's nothing wrong with them, just like there's nothing wrong with our thinking. Minds are meant to think. The strip of vertical blind in front of our faces doesn't mean anything about the view outside.

By understanding the nature of the blinds between us and our life, we can take them less seriously and less personally.

Chapter 20

Soda Story, Part 2

Okay, I promised you the second part of the soda story. This is where things get even more interesting.

I came home that day from the grocery store, minus my cans of soda, feeling very pleased with myself and really encouraged about the direction my habits, or, at least one habit, was moving in. The next day, however, lunchtime rolled around and things fell apart. But that turned out to be a powerful doorway to learning more about myself, how we all work, and this understanding.

What happened was that the next day, I felt a *very* strong urge to have a can of soda with my lunch. The old urges were rearing their ugly heads. I felt that urgent, driving, almost shouting feeling within me that said, "I must have a soda at lunch today!"

Initially, I was really disappointed to feel that feeling, but almost immediately I began bargaining with myself (as we do). "Well, maybe just this one last time. Maybe I'm tired today and need the energy boost." I don't remember the exact words of the bargaining session, but I'm sure you're pretty familiar with how that feels and sounds. So off I went to the corner store and bought one can of soda.

"Tomorrow, I'll for sure not have one," I said to myself after lunch.

Wrong.

The next day came and the same thing happened. Argh! Off I went to the corner store and bought one more can.

Day three. Same thing. Frustrating! "What is going on?!" I lamented to myself. "I thought I was done with this."

And then, later on day three, it occurred to me why this was happening: my brain was simply stuck in a rut. There was a neural pathway firing in response to the action of making lunch that was saying "Lunch = soda."

I reflected on this, and, given what I was learning about the changeable nature of my thinking, I bet myself that if I felt that urge the next day at lunch, it was possible that I could simply notice it and then it would pass.

That's exactly what happened.

Day Four dawned, and at noonish I started to think about preparing lunch. And sure enough, as soon as I had those thoughts, the old thoughts and urges about soda came bubbling up (so to speak).

"One more time!" my mind said. "Just for today, treat yourself. Come on, you can give up the habit tomorrow. Wouldn't you like just one last taste of your special treat before you say goodbye?"

But because I had learned about the moment-to-moment nature of thought, I was, on that day, able to hear those voices and feel those feelings and not obey them. I went about the business of toasting my bagel, or whatever, and by the time I got my lunch onto the plate and was walking into the living room to eat it, the voices and urges were gone. Like a marching band in a parade, they had moved their noisy selves down the block and had been replaced by whatever I was thinking about next.

And that was it. The soda spell was broken.

Epilogue

I feel it's important to share an addendum to the soda story. That story is not a representation of how all habits disappear. And it's not even a suggestion about a technique to use when dealing with the drive to overeat (i.e., surfing urges).

Rather, what it points to is that the changes to my soda habit came about insightfully. At no point did I use willpower to force myself to stop drinking soda. (After all, I'd tried that approach for years and it didn't work.) In the grocery store, the wisdom of my body led the way, letting me know it wasn't interested in soda any longer.

And then, a few days later, the way I dealt with the recurring urge at lunchtime was born out of curiosity. I wondered about what was happening and then got curious about an aspect of the inside-out understanding that I'd read and heard about—the changeable nature of our thinking—and decided to experiment to see what would happen.

In part 3 we'll dive deeper into the discussion about the vitally important role wisdom and insight play in this new paradigm, particularly when it comes to healing the drive to overeat.

Chapter 21

The Sky, Part 3

Imagine you're in your favorite place in your home, doing something you love. Maybe you're in your favorite reading chair, enjoying a good book. Maybe you're in the kitchen creating a meal for your family to enjoy.

You start to hear a noise, like someone is tapping their nails on a desk, only it's louder and more insistent. Curious, you lift your head and look around. What could that sound be? It's a rapid patter now, and getting louder. You wander away from what you were doing, following the sound. It gets louder as you approach a window. You look outside and realize it's hailing. There are hailstones hitting the window, and that's what you've been hearing. If they're large stones, they can make quite a racket.

You have a name for what's going on now: hail. And you have an understanding about how hail works: it is a weather phenomenon where little ice-like balls fall dramatically from the clouds in the sky.

And the hail, you realize, is crushing the plants in your garden. Or, if you live in Australia where everything seems to be more dangerous and exciting, the hailstones are so large they're denting your car, which is parked on the street. What a pain. You don't like the hail. It's causing problems.

Because of those problems and inconveniences (poor plants!), I'll make this one simple request of you: make the hail stop.

I often see that when people begin to grasp what this inside-out understanding is pointing toward, one of the first questions they'll have goes something like this: "If I understand that my thoughts and feelings are coming from inside me, rather than from my outside circumstances, then why have I been in a bad mood for three days? I can see my bad mood for what it is. Why won't it change?"

Your mood, good or bad, brief or long-lasting, is just like that hailstorm. You can name it and know it for what it is, but that doesn't mean you can make it stop.

However, you are also now aware that, just like that hailstorm, your mood will shift on its own.

There's nothing you need to do, or can do, about the hail. It's going to last as long as it lasts and then it will stop. The sun may come out after that, or it may rain, or it may snow. Who knows?

What the sky knows is that the weather is moving through it. Weather is temporary, always moving, and it does not affect the sky.

Part Three

Wisdom and Insight

Chapter 22

Looking Toward Wholeness

Never broken. Nothing lacking.

— Dr. Bill Petit

Did you know you can plant a tulip bulb (and other kinds of bulbs) upside down, and when the bulb starts to grow it will turn and head upward so that it can poke its head out of the soil? How does the bulb know how to do that? There, deep within the dark soil, how does the flower bulb know which way is up?

Did you know that trees communicate with one another, creating a vast underground network to offer healing, sustenance, and support to each other?[1]

How do butterflies, hummingbirds, and whales know the route to take on their migratory journeys? How does your skin know what to do in order to heal a cut? How do baby birds know when and how to peck their way out of the egg? You might say instinct, and that's true, but what is instinct and where does it come from?

These questions point out that there is an energy, a creative force, an intelligence, that powers the world and the universe we live in.

This same force spins the planets and keeps the Earth orbiting the sun. When a sunflower seed is planted, it knows it's supposed to grow up to be a sunflower and not an oak tree. This intelligent energy also exists in the microorganisms in our gut that keep our human digestive system working.

This energy source is far outside of our human control. We humans, with our big problem-solving brains, think we control and are the masters of so much. The reality is we're actually in control of very little. You don't beat your heart or breathe your lungs or turn the food you eat into energy. That all just happens. It's *amazing*, and whenever I take a step back from my busy thoughts and remember this, I am in awe, to say the least.

We can call this energy whatever we want. We could call it nature, or The Force, or life energy, or God, or universal energy, or Norman. It doesn't actually matter what it's called: it exists with or without a label. With or without us noticing it.

When we're caught up in our daily lives and our own human problems and challenges, we can be blind to the fact that this intelligence exists. I know I was, for roughly 50 years.

Chapter 23

The Hedgehog

Michael Neill, who teaches about this understanding, has a blog post on his website about the wisdom of the hedgehog. He explains that there's a line from a Greek poem by Archilochus (who? I have no idea) that says, "The fox knows many things, but the hedgehog knows one big thing."

In the post, Michael says this: "While foxes might be cunning and able to devise hundreds of strategies for catching unsuspecting hedgehogs off guard and eating them for dinner, the hedgehog has only one defensive strategy: to curl up in a ball, spiky spines exposed, and wait until the fox (or other predator) gives up and goes away."[1]

We humans often act more like that fox than we do the hedgehog. We use our big problem-solving brains to devise all kinds of strategies and tactics to fix ourselves and our problems. We can jump from one thing to another, frantically searching for answers, especially when something like the drive to overeat is bothering us. I know that was certainly my approach for decades.

But what Michael and the inside-out understanding are pointing to with the hedgehog parable is that we are more likely to be successful in life when we make a practice of doing the one thing that serves us really well: turning toward our own innate wisdom.

Instinct, insight, wisdom; whatever you want to call it, we all have it. Yet so often we don't trust that our own deep knowing about things is our best gauge for how to proceed in life.

The experience I shared earlier of going to the Equus workshop is an expensive example of what happens when we look outside ourselves for answers about how to end the drive to overeat. When we instead turn toward the wisdom that lies within each of us, our questions are answered insightfully. The understanding we experience via those insights is specific to each of us as individuals. Not that there's anything wrong with doing fun things like spending a few days in Southern California with a bunch of horses, but when it came to knowing how to heal my drive to overeat, what eventually worked was learning how to turn toward and listen to my own innate wisdom and insight. Just like that hedgehog.

Chapter 24

Insight and the Beach Ball

hy does insight matter in this exploration? Well, the way I see it, the drive to overeat (or any unwanted habit) is like a beach ball, and you're in the water, on top of that ball, trying to submerge it. Traditional approaches to curbing an overeating habit offer us strategies and tactics to cope with the ball's buoyancy and keep it under the water: straddling the ball is equal to tracking food points; pressing down hard on the ball is like using willpower to stay away from our favorite foods. It takes a tremendous amount of energy to keep that ball under the water. And the entire time we're doing this, the ball is fighting us because it's the nature of anything inflated with air to rise to the surface of a body of water. The laws of physics won't have it any other way.

We've all had the experience of starting a new diet or eating plan and having success for a day or two, only to have a loss of resolve and willpower defeat us. We take our attention off that metaphorical beach ball for even a second and it pops right back up to the surface. How many times have you had this happen to you? I can easily say hundreds.

I know this now: every traditional approach to eating is simply a redesigned or repackaged approach to keeping the beach ball under the water. Conversely, the understanding that we're exploring in this book, and that I explore in my work as a coach, instead uses insight to gradually deflate the beach ball.

When we look in this direction, every time we have an insight about our true nature, the nature of thought, and how all human beings work, the beach ball deflates a little. Eventually, all those insights add up and the ball is deflated completely, floating away on the tide. (Hopefully it was made of biodegradable material.) There's no longer anything to manage or try to control.

There is no prescribed set of insights, by the way. Your insights are going to be unique and meaningful to you. But whatever they are, they are going to universally have the same effect on the beach ball. That's the way insight works; the content or message or meaning of your insight is specific to you. Insight is a natural part of being human, and it is universal to all humans.

There's something else about this beach ball metaphor I'd like to bring up. Remember how I said that the inflated beach ball is obeying the laws of physics when it continually tries to float to the surface of a body of water? It can't *not* do that. If someone plonked the Sydney Opera House on top of that ball, it would still want to rise to the surface of the water. It would wiggle and squirm and eventually find a way to do what nature designed it to do.

Your drive to overeat is exactly the same.

It is going to keep rearing up, keep showing up, until you see it for what it is: a call to recognize your true nature. As Mavis Karn says, you are divinely engineered in this way. It's not a mistake that you feel the drive to overeat. It's not a failing or a weakness on your part. It's how you were designed. The cravings you experience are simply a message, like the little red circle on your phone that tells you you have a voice mail or text message. "Hey," it says, "no judgment here, but you've momentarily forgotten who you are. You've forgotten that you are entirely whole and innately well."

It wouldn't make sense if you got angry and judged yourself every time your phone let you know you have a voice mail message. That little red dot is simply doing its job.

So are your cravings.

When it comes to changing our eating habits, we've all been taught that more *doing* is the answer. But when we slow down and, to go back to an earlier metaphor, stop shaking up that snow globe, my experience has been that we become more aware, insightfully, of what is true about our overeating habit.

Culturally speaking, we are all so used to massive amounts of *doing* that this approach of relying on insight can seem wildly out of step with how we usually create change. However, from personal experience I can say that relying on insight is the *only* thing that has made a difference to my drive to overeat. Until I saw, insightfully, several truths about that drive and myself and my innate well-being, it didn't shift at all. Adding more techniques and strategies to try to eliminate the drive and control my food intake was just finding new ways to manage the beach ball.

It never worked.

Insight is what changed me from someone who felt over-taken by the drive to overeat for 30+ years to someone who is actually interested in eating well, who doesn't feel that drive any longer, and who is losing weight.

Chapter 25

More Thinking

I f you've tried to conquer the drive to overeat with logic and willpower, you probably learned what a poor strategy that is. Likely more than once. (I'm raising my hand and saying 'Me too!')

And I bet you've also had the experience of seeing something insightfully. One of those experiences where suddenly a truth dawns on you, and, in one instant, everything is changed. Maybe it was about a relationship or a situation you were in. Whatever it was, you know that 'Ah- ha!' feeling that I talked about in the previous chapter. And you also know that when you have one of those moments, you can't go back to un-seeing the thing you saw.

Conversely, when we try to 'fix' or heal the drive to overeat with logic and willpower, what we're really doing is layering a bunch of thinking onto an already existing pile of thoughts. That's like trying to dig a hole by throwing more dirt in the hole.

Not applying thinking to a problem can seem illogical to us and our big problem-solving brains. After all, that's how we solve problems like how to fix a flat tire or how to mend a hole in a sweater. It's how we've been taught to tackle most problems in life: apply some thinking to the situation and you'll come up with a solution.

However, when we take a step back, we can easily see that all that thinking hasn't fixed the growing problem of a population with expanding waistlines. If the traditional willpower- and deprivation-based weight loss approach worked, it would *work*. People like you and me wouldn't return again and again to try another system or another four-point plan only to fail and gain back the weight we'd lost, plus five pounds.

If thinking and willpower were the only things at play in your quest to stop the drive to overeat, you would have figured out how to do that *years* ago. You're a smart person. You desperately want to be free of the overeating yoke around your neck. You've thought about this problem so much that if we strung your thoughts together like a popcorn chain, they'd likely reach to the moon and back.

More thinking doesn't change the things we struggle with. Understanding does. Relying on insight and wisdom like the hedgehog does is what creates change.

Chapter 26

Willpower Is Not the Tool You Need

We think that safety comes through control and actually it comes through connection.

— Emily Rose Anderson

The reason willpower doesn't work when we're trying to deal with the drive to overeat is that the drive is trying to tell us something. In a previous chapter, we talked about how our feelings are a perfect feedback loop, letting us know that we're caught up in thinking that doesn't serve us. So, when we apply willpower to try to deal with the drive to overeat, it's like trying to hold back the tide with a beach towel.

Our bodies are wise and they know what they're doing. But a body doesn't have a voice, ironically, even though there is a voice box right there in your throat. The wisdom in your body can't sit you down and say, "Look, here's what's going on. You're caught up in a misunderstanding about how life works and how *you* work. Let me clear things up for you."

Instead, it has to communicate with you via your feelings, including the drive to overeat.

We curse that drive. Don't I know it! We rue the day it ever reared its head and lament that if only that drive would disappear, everything would be fine.

When a baby cries, there's a reason: it's hungry or tired. Its diaper is full. It has pain somewhere. Your drive to overeat is the same. It wants your attention. But contrary to what the old psychological paradigm advises, it's not saying there are old wounds you need to heal so that you can be free of the drive. It's saying that you're not seeing that you *are* healed. You *are* whole. There's nothing lacking in you, and there never was.

So, applying willpower to the drive to overeat is like trying to drink tea using a croquet mallet. No matter how well-intentioned you are, it's just not going to work. You're using the wrong tool for the job.

I'm pretty sure you know this. No doubt you've tried to apply willpower to your drive to overeat numerous times. The sad part is that when it didn't work, you blamed yourself. (I know I did.) So we try, again and again, and fail, over and over, innocently trying to drink tea with that croquet mallet.

Chapter 27

Boot Camps Don't Create Transformation

I'm not a reality TV watcher. Those programs are just not my cup of tea. But years ago, I recall watching a portion of a reality program about weight loss. I don't remember which one it was. It might have been British. But what I do remember is the follow-up story of the person who'd 'won' the competition.

The program was one that combined weight loss with a makeover for the participants. The contestants had coaching (both physical and psychological) and guidance and accountability up the wazoo, and when they'd lost the extra weight they were carrying, they were given a clothing makeover. A new, stylish wardrobe to fit their new bodies.

I didn't watch the whole season of this particular show, but I somehow caught an episode that was filmed months after the contest part of the program had ended. The producers were interviewing the man who'd won that season. And, no surprise to you or me, the weight he'd lost was coming back on. In fact, he confessed to the producers that it had started to come back on *before* the final episode of the show had been filmed. The new pants they'd chosen for him to wear during his big reveal were, he said, really tight on the day of shooting, and he wasn't sure he'd be able to button them up. I seem to recall him talking about eating all the chocolate bars and candy in the mini-fridge in his hotel room, but the clarity of that detail has been dulled by time.

The thing that stuck with me was that this fellow had likely experienced something those of us with the drive to overeat are intimately familiar with. Initially, the rush of euphoria about the support he was going to receive regarding changing his eating habits probably carried him along for a time. But what I suspect he discovered in the end was that he hadn't actually experienced transformation on the inside. Once those external cues and props were gone, he was still trying to keep the beach ball under the water.

When we are transformed from the inside, however, we *can't* go back to the way we were previously. It's just not possible.

This kind of transformation occurs when we turn our attention in the direction of our innate wellness and our wholeness rather than toward what's 'wrong' with us. When we insightfully see that the drive to overeat isn't pointing out our faults and that it is, in fact, pointing out how perfectly we are designed, we are transformed.

As I said before, the beach ball gradually begins to deflate until we no longer need to do anything to manage it.

Chapter 28

Suffering Is Optional

You can have your experience without your experience having you.

— Linda Pransky

I t seems to me that there is a sublime intelligence behind our human design. As aspects of the universe, we are here not to suffer, but to experience life. When we understand that experiences are just that—experiences—and that it is our thinking about them that causes us stress, we can then have a really difficult or hurtful experience without letting it have us. I'm not saying that life doesn't hand us each some really shitty moments. Of course it does. We're all going to experience pain and loss and even trauma, but when we know that at our home base, our essence, our default is peace and well-being, we can have those experiences and then let them float on down the river.

I say this as someone who has never had any kind of mystical or magical moment of touching the face of God or feeling utterly loved and blissed-out in a powerful meditation. I have a few friends who have had that sort of experience, and I used to think that it was a requirement for developing an understanding of my own true nature as peace and well-being. I thought that those kinds of experiences would be like a touchstone that I could remember and recall when I felt un-peaceful and unwell. But it turns out that's not the case.

I'm just a slob on the bus (to misquote Joan Osborne), and like everyone else, I muddle through each day, sometimes caught up in my thinking, sometimes not. Simply turning my attention toward the possibility that I am whole and well rather than broken and in need of fixing has opened a door that I didn't even realize was closed. Now I can feel the sunlight pouring in, and even when I can't feel it, I know it's there. Always. That feeling of warm sunlight on my face after a cold winter is who I am. And it is who you are.

Chapter 29

Getting Back Home

What you seek is with you and has been with you always.

— Sydney Banks

As I've mentioned, I'm a recovering self-help junkie. In the past, if someone offered me a strategy or tactic that promised to 'heal' me (and my overeating habit), I'd get onboard in a heartbeat. And when I used those strategies and tactics, as well-meaning as they were, the implication was that I was creating something out of nothing. For example, using mindfulness to observe my thinking and therefore be more present in the moment. Or using self-compassion to create a feeling of peace where I assumed there was an absence of peace. Or weighing and measuring my food, or counting food 'points' or calories as a way of managing and controlling the drive to overeat.

Conversely, what I've seen as I learn more about this inside-out understanding is that I don't need to create peace within myself because it's already there. I don't need to be mindful in order to be in the present moment because my mind will settle and return to the present moment naturally. And I don't need to control or manage what I eat because I naturally and innately have a desire to eat in a healthy way. That desire has been there all along, although it's been covered up by a lot of misplaced thinking about my being broken.

In the self-help realm, we are all so used to adding more strategies and tactics on top of our already sped-up thinking that it can be uncomfortable to begin to see that the answer lies in doing less, not more.

Years ago, I used to follow a self-help guru, and even took coach training from her, until I realized her approach to self-help and healing was causing me to feel more overwhelmed and stressed, not less. Her books were filled with so many strategies and tactics for managing life and controlling feelings that I ended up feeling like, on top of all my other problems, I was now juggling all the strategies and tactics I was learning, trying to remember which one to use in any given situation, and was left exhausted by it all. This guru's intentions were good, but unfortunately her approach left me feeling agitated, not peaceful.

Unlike in baseball, we never leave the 'home base' that is our innate peace and well-being. We might forget about it or get distracted from it, but it is never not there. And we don't need to do anything to get back there.

Seeing this makes all the difference when it comes to an overeating habit.

Part Four

The Beginning

Chapter 30

30 Years of Advice vs. Insight

You can't use an old map to find a new land.

— Gary Hamel

For 30+ years I took advice about how to lose weight and, I hoped, get rid of the drive to overeat. More than three decades. That's a *lot* of advice. And a lot of failure.

Advice is created because a tactic or strategy has worked well for the advice-giver. It's somewhat like offering a friend your very favorite food in the world—let's say that it is an ice cream sundae with colorful sprinkles and bananas and chocolate sauce with a cherry on top—and you're so excited to share this amazing masterpiece of flavors. But the person you're offering it to looks at you and says, "I'm allergic to dairy."

The ice cream sundae isn't for everyone.

What advice does is largely negate the innate wisdom and well-being of each person. There's the misunderstanding, the illusion that we are all living in that says we experience life from the outside in. And then, in addition to this, most advice points us in the wrong direction. Instead of pointing us inward, toward our own wisdom and knowing, it points us away from these things. As though those outside us know us better than we innately do, as though somehow, they are more connected to our own wisdom than we ourselves are. Granted, some of us (myself included) go through a lot of our lives being very disconnected from that innate wisdom; but 'good' advice points us inward, toward what we already have, rather than outward, toward what *they* have for us.

Now, it should go without saying that if we're talking about changing a tire or performing brain surgery, of course you're going to want to take advice and learn how to do those things. But in this chapter, I'm talking about a wholistic connection to that which exists beyond our thinking, and beyond our human experience.

When we turn our attention to what is true and universal for all humans, and away from the techniques or strategies that have worked for a few people, we begin to grow an awareness of how our human experience really works. And when we do this, we become more aware of the blue sky that is there surrounding us at every moment, even when we can't see it.

If advice worked, then I'd be the poster child for it. I've been swimming in a sea of advice about how to curb the drive to overeat for more than half my life. Sure, some of that advice was helpful momentarily. And maybe some of it has been very helpful for other people. But again, I say, if advice worked, we'd all be cured of our overeating habits. There's SO much advice out there in the diet industry. If that approach worked, shouldn't it have worked on us by now?

Embracing the new psychological paradigm I've shared in this book will be a big leap for many. It flies in the face of everything we think we understand about how life works. But if you've made it this far in the book, you may have seen a glimpse of what I'm trying to point you toward. And a glimpse is all you need to begin turning in this direction.

You and I may be quite similar; you may have tried all the advice-giving books and courses and plans as well and ended up, just like me, still battling the drive to overeat and weighing more than you ever have. The suffering that comes with that experience is real.

The irony is that I can't tell you *how* your drive to overeat will change. Only you will experience that. This book is my way of showing you that there's a way other than diets and techniques for managing the overeating beach ball. Hopefully what I've shared has given you a glimpse of what's possible when we look toward our own innate wisdom and well-being.

Additionally, you may have gathered by now that even though this book is called *It's Not About the Food*, it could be called *It's Not About the Drinking* or *It's Not About the Spending*. The inside-out understanding points us toward how our human experience works in all circumstances, not just when it comes to overeating. This understanding points to how we work; therefore, it applies in any situation or circumstance. It relates to every area of our lives.

If you decide to continue learning about how we humans work from the inside out, you'll likely find that every area of your life will be affected for the better. I know I have. Yes, my eating habits have changed, my weight is dropping along with my blood pressure, and my relationships have also improved. I am far more patient and kind to myself and others. And the anxiety I used to feel pretty consistently has all but disappeared. I say this not to brag, but to be encouraging.

Remember my analogy about learning to play the guitar? If you've made it this far in this book, then you've learned to strum a chord or two.

Keep going—there're more to see. Keep listening. Keep reading. Keep exploring and questioning. The best thing you can do to find the peace you've been searching for is to stay in the conversation.

Want More Understanding?

As I mentioned early on, the exploration of this understanding is like learning a different language or learning to play a musical instrument. It can take some time to get our heads around the concepts and principles because they are generally the opposite of what we've been taught. It's a school of thought we're not usually very familiar with.

With that in mind, I've created a series of free videos to deepen your understanding. The Freedom From Overeating series further explores many of the ideas I've shared in this book and includes printable visual aids to remind you where to put your focus, and a list of recommended resources for further exploration. You can start watching those videos today at:

alexandraamor.com/start

Additionally, I host a weekly podcast called Unbroken, which you can subscribe to wherever you get your podcasts. Join me every Thursday when my guests and I explore the inside-out nature of being human and how we can all be more in touch with our innate wisdom, well-being, and peace of mind, specifically with an eye toward ending our habits. You can even submit your questions about anything you've read in this book for a Monday Q&A episode at alexandraamor.com/questions

If you would like one-on-one coaching about your overeating habit, I offer that as well. Learn more at:

alexandraamor.com/coaching

I look forward to connecting with you soon.

With love,

Alexandra

About the Author

Alexandra Amor is a lifelong explorer of what it means to be human.

For over 20 years Alexandra has been writing both fiction and non-fiction books, all with the themes of love, connection, and the search for understanding. She began her writing career with an Amazon best-selling, award-winning memoir about ten years she spent in a cult in the 1990s.

A former Vancouverite, Alexandra now lives in a magical fishing village on Vancouver Island and spends each day writing, exploring the inside-out understanding, and creating. When she's not doing that you'll likely find her walking on a beach or worrying that the vacuum cleaner feels ignored. In her spare time she serves on the boards of her local hospice association and seniors' independent living facility.

Learn more at AlexandraAmor.com

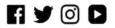

Also by Alexandra Amor

Memoir

Cult, A Love Story

Freddie Lark Mysteries

Lark Lost

Lark Underground

Historical Mysteries

Charlie Horse

Horse With No Name

The Outside of a Horse

Water Horse

The Horse You Rode In On

A One Horse Open Sleigh

Juliet Island Romantic Mysteries

Love and Death at the Inn

Children's Animal Adventure Novels

Sugar & Clive and the Circus Bear

Sugar & Clive and the Bank Robbery

Sugar & Clive and the Movie Star

Larry at the Wedding (A Sugar & Clive Novella)

Acknowledgments

Huge thanks to copyeditor Jennifer McIntyre whose brilliant editing work and incisive, always valuable feedback makes every book I write far better than I could ever manage alone. Jen, you are worth your weight in gold and I am so grateful for our working relationship!

Thanks also to the Tuesday mastermind group. You inspire me and remind me to keep looking toward wisdom for answers. I love you all.

Notes

22. Looking Toward Wholeness

1. Source: *Finding the Mother Tree*, by Suzanne Simard (Penguin Canada, 2021).

23. The Hedgehog

1. Source: https://www.michaelneill.org/cfts1135/